I0092777

COMPULSIVE LYING MASTERY: THE SCIENCE BEHIND WHY WE LIE AND HOW TO STOP LYING TO GAIN BACK TRUST IN YOUR LIFE

The Ultimate Cure Guide for Addiction to Simple White Lies to Compulsive or Pathological Lying Disorder, Sociopathy, and ASPD

DAVID WHITEHEAD

Silk Publishing

INTRODUCTION

"If you tell the truth, you don't have to remember anything."

— MARK TWAIN

Everyone lies from time to time. Maybe the reason for it is to avoid embarrassment, to avoid hurting the feelings of someone else, or for any other kind of reasoning with an innocent sheer. But some people keep lying habitually and intentionally. They tend to deceive others without any sort of remorse. Well, what they are suffering from is known as compulsive lying disorder. At times, the tendency to tell a lie gets so deeply entrenched in a compulsive liar's personality that all their lies tend to get interwoven with reality in a way that the person himself starts believing them.

In case you know someone with this disorder, or worse, if you are in a romantic or familiar relationship with one, it is pretty normal for you that the level of frustration will skyrocket whenever you can feel that you are being lied to.

Also, living with a compulsive liar might turn out to be dangerous emotionally. You won't be able to rely on or trust that person. So, can't anything be done to treat this disorder? Luckily, the answer is yes, and that is what this book is all about.

There are plenty of books on this subject on the market, thanks again for choosing this one! Every effort was made to ensure it is full of as much helpful information as possible; please enjoy!

WHAT IS COMPULSIVE LYING?

Compulsive lying is the chronic behavior of habitual lying. Unlike opting for white lies occasionally to prevent yourself from hurting the feelings of someone else or getting into serious trouble, a compulsive liar keeps lying for no specific reason at all. It might make it frustrating or challenging for you to ensure what to do if you come across such a person. Although compulsive lying has been recognized for many years now, there is still no clear definition for the condition. Compulsive lying for some people might result from certain mental illnesses, like antisocial personality disorder, while others might have the same without any known medical reason.

WHO IS A COMPULSIVE LIAR?

A compulsive liar is a person who keeps lying compulsively. While there might be a wide range of reasons behind compulsive lying, it is not yet clear who some people tend to lie this way. Some lies are told to make the person look like a hero or for gaining sympathy or acceptance, while there is nothing else to be gained from telling lies. It has been found from some evidence from the year 2007 that issues dealing with the central nervous system might predispose someone to compulsive lying. In fact, compulsive lying is also regarded as a trait of specific personality disorders, like an antisocial personality disorder. Head injuries or trauma might also play distinct roles in compulsive lying, in addition to some abnormality in the ratio of hormone-cortisol. A study from the year 2016 regarding what happens inside the brain when you lie figured out that the more number of untruths someone tells, the more frequent and more accessible their lying becomes.

The results of the study also indicated that self-interest might also fuel dishonesty. Although the study did not talk about compulsive lying in specific, it might provide us with particular insights regarding why compulsive liars tend to lie so much as they do. There are particular characteristics and traits that can define a compulsive liar. Let's have a look at them.

THEIR LIES DO NOT COME WITH ANY CLEAR BENEFIT

While any average person might opt for lying to avoid any kind of uncomfortable situation, like getting into severe trouble or an embarrassment, a compulsive liar might tell lies or stories that do not come with any sort of objective benefit. Family and friends might also find this thing very frustrating as the person who is lying does not stand to get anything from the lies.

THE STORIES TOLD ARE GENERALLY COMPLICATED, DRAMATIC, AND DETAILED

Compulsive liars can be great storytellers. All their lies tend to be extremely colorful and detailed. Even though above everything, compulsive liars can be very convincing.

THEY TEND TO PORTRAY THEMSELVES AS THE VICTIM OR THE HERO

Besides being made the victim or hero of their stories, compulsive liars tell lies that are generally geared toward gaining sympathy, admiration, or acceptance by other people.

THEY TEND TO BELIEVE THEIR LIES AT TIMES

A compulsive liar tells stories and lies that somewhere fall between delusion and conscious lying. They, at times, tend to believe their lies.

It is pretty challenging to know what can be done with a compulsive liar who might not be conscious of their lying. Some of the compulsive liars tend to do this so often that the experts believe they might not have any idea of the difference between fiction and fact after some point in time. Also, compulsive liars are natural performers. They are pretty eloquent and also know how they can engage the attention of others while speaking. They are original and creative, and quick thinkers who do not generally show any typical signs of lying, like avoiding eye contact or long pauses. When any question is thrown at them, they might start speaking a lot without being specific or answering the actual question.

COMPULSIVE LIES VS. WHITE LIES

Most human beings lie at some point or the other in their lives. It has been found from various research that we tend to tell approximately 1.75 lies daily. The majority of all such lies are considered to be 'white lies.' On the other hand, compulsive lies are told habitually and consistently. Most of the time, they tend to appear continuous and pointless.

WHITE LIES

White lies are generally occasional and are considered:

- Harmless
- Small fibs
- Without any kind of harmful intent
- Told to deal with the feelings of someone else or to avoid getting in some kind of trouble

Some of the examples of white lies are:

- Saying that you have got a bad headache for getting out of a meeting or a party

- Saying that you had already paid the electricity bill when in actuality you forgot to pay the same
- Lying about why you reached office late

COMPULSIVE LIES

Compulsive lies are generally:

- Continuous
- Told compulsively and frequently
- Told for no particular gain or reason
- Told for making oneself look like the victim or hero
- Not deterred by risk or guilt of getting caught

Some of the examples of compulsive lying are:

- Developing false history, like saying that they have experienced or achieved something that they have not
- Claiming to suffer from some sort of life-threatening illness that they do not have in actuality
- Opting for lies to impress someone else, like saying they are in touch with a famous person

COMPULSIVE LIARS AND SOCIOPATHY

A sociopath is someone who lies just to get their way out. A sociopath comes with very little concern for other people and can opt for anything to protect their interests.

Such individuals are generally focused on a goal, focused on lying, and can get things done in their way. It does not matter if their work gets done at the expense of others. Sociopaths come with no form of regard for other's feelings. They tend to get away with all that they do as they are generally charismatic and charming. But they put into use their charm for manipulating others and get what they want.

On the other hand, a compulsive liar is someone who comes with the habit of telling lies. Lying at times is normal and often acts as a simple reflexive way of responding to questions. Compulsive liars generally try to bend the truth, no matter small or large.

Compulsive liars face difficulties in telling the truth. Generally, they are not convinced by the fact, so they give their best to make up things and twist the actual truth as doing so only feels like the right thing for them. Compulsive lying might get developed right from early childhood, especially when someone is exposed to some kind of environment where it is necessary to tell lies. They are not much manipulative; however, they border on being manipulators.

IT CAN DEVELOP FROM CHILDHOOD

Admit it that you lie, and all of us do the same at some point in our lives. We all have lied; however, they are white lies. Did you ever lie to a close friend of yours regarding how they looked in the expensive dress they just bought? Did you ever tell a friend of yours that they are looking great even when it is not the case? How many times have you acted sick only because you felt lazy to opt for work or while going out somewhere with friends? No matter what the situation is that prompted you to opt for lies, you will need to accept that lying is a natural part of every human being. But when you permit all these white lies to keep piling up, the habit of lying might turn out to be habitual. It might slowly evolve into the disorder of compulsive lying. As already said earlier, compulsive lying might develop from childhood as well.

It tends to develop at times when more opportunities to lie are present in front of someone. Childhood lies are generally as simple as telling your mother that you are feeling sick and you do not want to go to school, or it might be a white lie to run away from getting punished for breaking the favorite vase of your mother. As one gets ahead in life, from childhood to adolescence and then to adulthood, telling lies becomes more frequent. Compulsive liars had the opportunity to experience having some sense of 'power' over situations, events, and even other people, as they tell lies. They might turn out to be uncomfortable and agitated when someone presses on them for telling the truth. When all of this turns into a daily habit, mental health experts can say that a person suffers from compulsive lying disorder.

CAUSES

Research is still going on, and the actual causes of compulsive lying are not known yet. It is not clear whether compulsive lying is a symptom of some other condition or is a condition in itself. But compulsive lying is a feature of various other states, like personality disorders or factitious disorder.

PERSONALITY DISORDERS

Compulsive lying might turn out to be a possible symptom of some personality disorders, like:

- NPD or narcissistic personality disorder
- BPD or borderline personality disorder
- APD or antisocial personality disorder

A borderline personality disorder is a condition that makes it challenging for the sufferer to keep their emotions under regulation. BPD people might experience excessive mood swings, feel great insecurity and instability, and not have any stable sense of themselves. The fundamental hallmarks of NPD are fantasies regarding immense importance and the need for special treatment or admiration. Researchers argue that compulsive lying might occur in all those suffering from APD; all those with this condition might lie for pleasure or personal gain. People suffering from NPD or BPD might lie for distorting the reality into something that can fit with all the emotions they are feeling, instead of the facts. Personality disorders of this nature might result in significant challenges in regards to interpersonal relationships.

FACTITIOUS DISORDER

Factitious disorder is a condition in which individuals act as if they are mentally or physically ill when in reality, they are not. Factitious disorder by proxy is when a person lies about someone else having some kind of illness. It is most common in mothers trying to feign illness in their children and lie to the doctor about the same. The exact causes behind the factitious disorder are not known, but the theories include:

- Childhood neglect or abuse
- Genetic or biological causes
- Low level of self-esteem
- Depression
- The presence of any personality disorder
- Substance abuse

ARE YOU A COMPULSIVE LIAR?

Compulsive lying might start small. The lies can become more dramatic and elaborate with time, especially if needed to cover up for a complete life. They tend to get complicated with an unnecessary amount of details. All those who tend to lie frequently are not compulsive liars. One of the most distinguishing features of a compulsive lie is that it does not come with a motive. So, an individual who keeps exaggerating stories frequently for making themselves look more exciting and keeps lying for covering up all the mistakes made by them is not likely to be compulsive lying. Compulsive lies are pretty easy for other people to verify, which might ultimately be harmful to the individual who keeps telling them. For instance, the person might opt for false accusations or grand claims regarding their past that are pretty easy for others to be checked.

Are you a compulsive liar? Well, some sure signs and symptoms will ensure whether you are a compulsive liar or not.

SIGNS AND SYMPTOMS

Let's have a look at some of the signs and symptoms that can indicate whether someone is a compulsive liar or not.

UNNECESSARY DISHONESTY

A person who is a compulsive liar will keep telling lies regarding everything, even when that person cannot benefit from hiding the truth. Also, the intensity of lying is quite frequent. For example, a compulsive liar can opt to fabricate stories regarding the most trivial things, such as their favorite color or snack. The majority of the time, as you ask them a question, he/she will answer automatically with a lie. It does not even matter if there is a logical reason why they opt for a dishonest answer. Compulsive liars do not come with any intent to lie or hurt; however, they do so anyway. You can say that it takes place almost instantaneously. It is more or less like lying is an integrated part of their overall system that they can never run away from. Frequent lies might result in strained relationships, specifically for the liar who fails to keep track of their lies.

In case you feel the same with yourself, you might be suffering from compulsive lying disorder. You will have to be attentive to the lies you opt for to determine your condition.

LOOKING FOR ATTENTION

Compulsive lying disorder might develop during early childhood, often because of the desire of the child to get attention from their parents, other kids, or caregivers. Children tend to come with various forms of wild imagination, and they would opt for the fabrication of fascinating stories and thus soliciting disbelief from everyone present around them. The majority of parents try to brush off all such stories as children are generally creative, so they try to dismiss them as passing fancy. According to most parents, their kids would 'outgrow' such habits eventually. But if the lies get tolerated, children would start assuming that is something acceptable that they can do. They might think that fabricating stories only to get others like them is entirely okay. Most parents cannot realize that their children's lying behavior can go on until they become adults.

FABRICATION OF STORIES FOR BEING SUPERIOR

Compulsive liars tend to believe that they deserve to always be the center of attraction. They just love to think that they are superior to others, and they opt for the fabrication of stories so that others look up to them. They desire others to put them on a pedestal. According to them, the best way of getting the attention of others is to fabricate stories regarding themselves, their capabilities, their achievements, and all those extraordinary things that they can do. All such stories are only intended for providing them with a hero image. But there is a definite drawback that comes with this very practice. When others find out the truth eventually, they are most likely to be held in contempt, and others will indeed dislike them.

When such a thing happens, compulsive liars tend to lie even more so that they can just shake off being known as deceivers and liars.

When an individual suffering from compulsive lying disorder becomes an adult, all their outrageous stories tend to get more grounded. However, even if they are filled with exceptional skills, accomplishments, and talents.

LIES FOR COVERING UP

Compulsive liars need to give extra attention to keep others under the control of their deception. But there are rare times when their shield of lies tends to unravel, and the true nature gets exposed. When such a thing happens, they immediately put back the walls and start lying even more to rebuild their images. The majority of the time, they would opt to tell elaborate stories, such as being accused falsely and developing more stories to prove that they are innocent. In fact, they might try to discredit all those individuals who unwrapped their true nature. But the truth has to come out, and when a compulsive liar gets caught in any form of predicament, they will get forced to tell the truth. However, the compulsive liar might wriggle himself/herself out effectively out of the mess and reclaim their place eventually.

STORY STEALING AND PRESENTING THEM AS THEIR OWN

Any compulsive liar will have several role models from whom they get all their stories. Plagiarism can be considered the key to living a life that any compulsive liar wants to attain. They can easily take away stories that they heard from someone else or stories of their loved ones or friends and label all such stories as their very own. In case they fail to find something interesting from others present around them, there are several TV and movie plotlines for them to adapt. Compulsive liars tend to give their all for not allowing the stories to fall apart as they are scared of being found out. They would most likely weave all their magic around all those people who are unsuspecting. In most cases, compulsive liars tend to start believing their fabricated stories as their very reality.

CONTENT SEEKING RESPECT FROM OTHERS

Compulsive liars are most likely to suffer from low self-esteem. So, they try to resort to the development of stories that are not true to make themselves feel better. They want others to regard them as high achievers. As they do not possess anything to present as proof, they try to concoct various stories of their greatness, in turn, trying to believe that they are great indeed.

CHARACTERISTICS OF COMPULSIVE LIARS

Whenever it comes to the context of compulsive lying, there are six definite characteristics that can make sure whether someone is suffering from compulsive lying disorder or not. It can be used for yourself as well.

- **They tend to study others around them:** According to mental health experts, compulsive liars opt for studying others who are present around them so that they can take full advantage of all those people. The majority of the time, compulsive liars would not want others to determine the truth. They make it a point to learn in detail about others: their interests, beliefs, and various other factors, so that they can be persuaded without much effort.

- **They do not feel empathetic:** It might be quite hard to believe, but it is the only truth. Compulsive liars come with little to no form of regard for the feelings of other people. They do not tend to pause and try to think about what the other person might be feeling in response to all their lies. It can be said that there is no presence of the word 'empathy' in their vocabulary.

- **They do not experience guilt:** Any regular or occasional liar comes with a sense of consciousness. Whenever others stop asking questions or just change the topic, they tend to feel relieved. But for compulsive liars, they do not care to showcase any form of emotion while uttering a lie. An average liar would get stressed out whenever presented with a question for their statement. Compulsive liars tend to remain unfazed when they get confronted with an array of questions.

- **They do not do those things that they are perceived to do:** Compulsive liars do not do ordinary things that they are generally expected to do, such as touching their nose, being fidgety, or shifting from one seat to another at the time of lying. They tend to be relaxed, can make eye contact, and also show no form of emotion.
- **They might be manipulative and sneaky:** A majority of the time, they know what needs to be done and what to say to believe in their lies.
- **They show unusual behaviors:** Can you remember how nervous you were at the time of telling a white lie? It is pretty standard for you as you would not want to get caught. The majority of compulsive liars tend to develop their lying skills from childhood, and as they reach adulthood, lying turns out to be second nature for them. They would rarely showcase discomfort. However, when others try to call them out for lying or get confronted, they try to get defensive and agitated. All their anger results in more lies to cover up their old lies.

DIAGNOSIS

Compulsive lying is not like any other formal diagnosis. However, a mental health expert or a therapist can easily recognize the related behaviors as signs of any other underlying condition, like factitious disorder or personality disorder. All these disorders include several overall symptoms, besides compulsive lying. People who are suffering from these conditions also showcase other signs. It is also possible for compulsive lying to be a free and independent symptom. Some people get indulged in compulsive lying without any form of an underlying medical condition. It might be a challenge for therapists or mental health experts to determine whether someone is suffering from compulsive lying disorder. There are no biological or pathological tests for the same. To diagnose most of the mental health issues, therapists opt for clinical interviews. In case the person is not honest regarding their habit of lying, it might be necessary for the therapist or mental health expert to talk to his/her family members or close friends to identify the patterns of compulsive lying.

❧ 3 ❧

REASONS TO STOP LYING

Truth does not come with several versions. The truth might come with various sides to it. It might be complex or complicated to understand; however, it does exist in one single performance. But still, the majority of us tend to struggle with the same. Some of us might not be outright liars, just like compulsive liars, but we try to shade the truth to make it fit more comfortably into our daily lives. We try to do so to keep it away from disrupting anything from our relationships to our careers to our daily afternoons. People tend to lie in one out of five of their daily interactions – found in a recent study. There are things that are pretty essential to consider – How honest is the world that we have tried to create all around ourselves? How much or how often do we tell lies to ourselves? On the flip side, do we try to intimidate other people in ways that might also make them hide the truth?

It is quite a normal and expected thing for people to bring out only those parts of the truth that they think are acceptable or make up what their people would like to hear, leaving the actual fact hidden behind. They might lie by omission or opt for white lies that come with the power of painting a whole different picture of reality. The lies told by compulsive liars also tend to do the same, or maybe more than that. Compulsive liars tend to change the entire picture without even trying to keep a portion of the same intact. No matter what kind of lie it is, it is no surprise that all such lies do not only hurt relationships but they can also destroy them outright. Even lies that are told for protecting others might leave you with a bad feeling if you are a white liar. It will provide you with an unauthentic sense. However, it is not the same with compulsive liars in this regard.

Let's look at some of the ways people tend to lie and how all of that can hurt the various areas of life.

HOW DO PEOPLE LIE AND HOW DO THEY HURT?

There are various ways in which people of today tend to lie. But they also hurt their lives in specific ways.

RESPONSE CONTROLLING

When you converse with a close friend about any interaction with your lover or a colleague, do you tend to only tell your side of the entire story? Do you try to leave out a tiny but essential detail regarding something you just brought to the table? Do you try to rephrase the not-so-desirable words that you said at that moment? Try to give it a thought that all such subtle changes might influence the response and attitude of your friend. Are you just trying to make your friend say what you want to hear? Right in the end, how true is their overall response in case you tried to manipulate the outcome strategically?

As you try to control any response simply by hiding the truth behind you, you tend to develop an alternate and agreed-upon world between the other person and you. You might start getting advice that might be simply based on false information. Also, you will deny yourself the integrity and value that someone else's actual opinions might have helped you.

LYING BY OMISSION

Have you ever tried to complain to someone that you are not being able to lose weight without mentioning the giant burger you just downed for your afternoon snack? All of us have times when we try to leave out the less desirable details. At times, we tend to do this for being sensitive or to spare someone else's feelings. But sometimes, all such details matter, and we all know the same. For instance, when your partner asks about your day, you might not try to mention how you bumped into your ex and had lunch together. Or maybe you are trying to conceal a current flirtation with a colleague of yours. All such acts might not seem like deception on your part. However, try to imagine how your life partner would view them.

No matter whether there is nothing to shade or anything real that you would not want others to know about, trying to leave out essential facts might make you feel shady only if you are not a compulsive liar. It might create a hotbed for future deceptions. On the contrary, developing a kind of environment where you can be free about all such things will help promote a feeling of honest communication and mutual trust.

EXAGGERATION

The insecurities of people regarding themselves might result in them trying to hide a particular image of themselves. They might experience a requirement of approval from other people. But whenever you try to exaggerate or do not present the honest version of yourself, you will be left feeling like a fraud, which might also hurt your self-esteem in the future. There exists a fine line between focusing on your attributes and inflating your abilities completely. You might just promise to get done with some work at the office that you are well aware of not completing on time. You might even exaggerate to your senior when it comes to the context of your skill level or progress. Trying to do so will most likely result in trouble as your actions will surely fail to match the words.

Sometimes, you might take the help of lies to compensatefor your guilt. For instance, parents often tend to do this with their children – for example, missing a football game and then promising that they will show at every game for the remaining season, which only results in disappointment very soon. It is pretty difficult to hide a missed meeting, broken trust or promise, or a not-so-good performance. Exaggerating will make you look untrustworthy. All your words will start meaning much less when the actual reality does not tend to match. Additionally, you might never come to believe that you are being selected or cared for being who you are.

PROTECTION

People are often trained by their inner critic not to directly express all they feel for other people. You might have set up a guard that directs you not to be vulnerable. You might try to downplay all your emotions or just start acting like you do not even care, as you would not want to look or feel like a fool. However, trying to defend yourself using false portrayals or deceptions of who you genuinely are might drive you away from all your goals. It will also stop you from attaining what you want in life.

COVERT COMMUNICATION OR GOSSIP

Gossip can be regarded as an epidemic. It can be found in every household, workspace, coffee house, and any possible place. It can be taken as a booming industry that has all the control over media. One of the biggest problems with talking about someone right behind their back is that you might flat out deny all such observations when you come face-to-face with that very person. You can quickly figure out how all of this might turn out to be harmful to all your relationships. A loving partner or a close friend should be the one with whom you can talk openly, offer your feedback, and get back the same from them. Also, gossip gives birth to cynicism and might also destroy compassion. It is a devastating way of dealing with the actual observations indirectly. When you opt for straightforward communication in place of gossip, you can turn out to be more compassionate, genuine, appealing, and a person to have around.

Some people tend to believe that lying is necessary for surviving in a relationship. Well, that is not true at all. Trying to mislead someone distorts the reality and often makes them go crazy, which can be regarded as one of the wicked things that can be done to someone else. So, what can be done to be honest? Well, you can start being honest with your self. Shading the actual truth often comes from abiding by the inner critical voice that never stays on your side, directs you to opt for protection by telling you various things like people will only accept you if you try not to reveal yourself. For your boss, it might tell you, "You have been messing things up lately, so tell your boss that you have solved all the problems on your own without anyone's help." For your spouse, it might say, "Do not tell her that you do not remember the anniversary; it might result in a fight." Getting to know the inner critic will help separate you from the real point of view and start acting against it.

You can start taking chances on all those you care about by being more direct and honest with them. The truth might not be that easy to hear all the time; however, you can earn a considerable amount of respect and trust from all those whose opinions matter to you in the long term. When it is about the truth, it is essential to think about whether you want others to trust you. Is there any value of integrity in your life, and you want all your words reflect in the actions? Committing to all such attributes on the level of behavior will allow you to live an honest life and have open communications.

CAN LYING HELP YOU WIN IN THE LONG-TERM?

Well, the answer to this is no. Lying for gaining more indicates that you do not have enough. So, you have to cheat for gaining something that you do not have in the first place. In the long-term, doing so will repel all those people away from you who might help you succeed. As you lie, it will make you look ugly and selfish together. There are no shortcuts in life. As human beings, we all are wired to stay away from all those people who lie. Deep inside, all of us just hate to be presented with lies. Well, you will get caught eventually. The only way in which you can progress in life is with the truth. Truth can help you set free from:

- Failures
- Lack of fulfillment
- Feeling dreadful about lying
- Opting for the wrong thing
- Not being the person who you really are

OTHER BENEFITS OF NOT LYING

While most of us are not compulsive liars, all those small white lies add up quickly and tend to change the patterns of our behaviors. It tends to make us more judgmental and suspicious. However, the bigger problem comes from all those lies that just gnaw at us regularly. Our habit of lying is connected to our health directly. So, not lying comes with several benefits related to our overall health.

- **Reduces stress:** Recent research has established a connection between frequent lying and enhanced risks of stress, anxiety, and depression. Stress acts as a precursor for various other chronic health problems, besides degrading our immunity, affecting our appetite, making us angry, feel tired, and more prone to headaches.
- **Boosts immunity:** We all have come across the saying, "No other medicine can be as effective as laughter." Having happy thoughts helps in the production of endorphins, which tend to make us feel good, besides supporting the functioning of our immunity system. As we lie, we have lots of things to deal with. All of that might result in worrying, which reduces the chances of experiencing endorphins that do good for our immunity.
- **Better sleep:** Deciding how to lie to others can keep you awake at night. Lying can make sleeping a difficult task and might even result in a bad nightmare. Also, lack of sleep results in weight gain, headache, and depression.
- **Better digestion:** Only a few things can make you feel sick in your stomach instantly as telling a big lie. Repeated lying can result in nausea, irritable bowel syndrome, stress eating, loss of appetite, and various other eating disorders.

- **Reduces the risk of cancer:** Although there are no studies that directly connect cancer and lying, there are prevailing connections between certain types of cancer and stress. As already discussed above, the less we tend to lie, the less will be the stress, which will help save our lives and make them enjoyable.

❧ 4 ❧
TREATMENTS FOR COMPULSIVE LYING DISORDER

Compulsive liars tend to lie without any specific reason. They just do so out of habit. The treatment process is considered to be a bit complicated; however, according to medical experts, it is possible. In case you are the one who needs treatment, you can expect the mental health expert to spend a great deal of time with the process of treatment to ensure that he/she gets access to all the required information for arriving at a proper diagnosis. The treatment options will depend on several factors - the sufferer themselves, their all-around health, and any underlying condition that they might need help with. The necessary treatments will mainly revolve around the modification of behavior along with various other things.

COUNSELING

The best available treatment option for compulsive lying disorder is counseling. Compulsive liars lie, and they will eventually accept that they lie; however, they cannot stop. The sessions of counseling will also try to diagnose various other underlying conditions too. Family therapy, couples therapy, or group therapy might be recommended by a therapist or a mental health expert. Let's have a look at them.

GROUP THERAPY AND HUMANISTIC THERAPY

While most psychodynamic therapists tend to concentrate on the patient's unconscious processes of the brain, humanistic therapists pay attention to the conscious experiences of the patients. There are certain similarities between humanistic therapy and psychotherapy. Both treatment options assume that the past of a person has a lot to do with their current behavior.

PERSON-CENTERED THERAPY

Carl Rogers developed the therapy. He believed that disorders like compulsive lying are the result of roadblocks that people experience in the path of self-actualization. According to Carl, compulsive liars might just start lying as they sought out some form of approval from the peers. So, they tend to wear a mask and start lying about who they are and all their experiences. Compulsive liars would eventually be aware of the inner voices and tend to develop a self-concept of distorted nature. As the final result, all such individuals start believing their lies. In person-centered therapy, an environment is created for compulsive liars where they can accept their true selves.

The therapy concept is non-directive, which indicates that the patient himself/herself will be the responsible one for leading the treatment progress rather than the therapist. In this therapy model, the therapist will keep rephrasing all those things expressed by the patient without any form of judgment. It will permit compulsive liars to explore all their feelings to bury underneath all their lies.

COGNITIVE THERAPY

Cognitive therapists can help compulsive liars determine and correct all their faulty attitudes and thinking, leading to their obsessive need to lie. There are various options available in this form of therapy.

- **Rational emotive behavioral therapy:**
  Some of the therapists believe that the lies developed by compulsive liars result from their irrational belief that they need to have the approval of all those present around them. Though it can be understood to desire the admiration of others, it is regarded to be irrational when someone starts thinking that he/she cannot just live without it. In rational emotive behavioral therapy, mental health experts of therapists dispute the patients' irrational beliefs and provide them with the needed help to develop certain alternative ideas. The concerned therapists will help compulsive

liars to find out more desirable outlets in place of lying.

- **Beck's cognitive therapy:** With the help of this therapy, compulsive liars are asked to determine and change all the errors that they have in their thinking. They might be asked to keep track of instances in which they felt the urge or need to lie. Therapists then try to dispute all their distorted thoughts and replace them with much more rational alternatives. Another form of cognitive therapy is creating a reality where patients can test their negative beliefs in real situations. For instance, if a compulsive liar tends to believe that no one would like him/her if they fail to create new stories, he/she can test out the theory, and call their close friends or family members and opt for telling a story that happened in actuality. In most cases, the concerned patient might feel surprised to see that others appreciate real stories much more than their lies.

- **Cognitive behavioral therapy:** In this form of therapy, therapeutic techniques are used to change the behaviors and thoughts of patients. CBT or cognitive behavioral therapy assumes that the alterations in the thinking patterns and beliefs of a person will result in desirable changes in their overall behavior. Therapists use various behavioral techniques to correct the ways of automatic thoughts that might trigger compulsive lying. CBT comes with some outstanding records of treating compulsive lying and various other emotional disorders, like socio-phobia, stress disorders, and personality disorders.

- **Eclectic therapy:** It uses various approaches for achieving therapeutic benefits. For instance, therapists might use behavioral therapy to entice changes in the behaviors of a compulsive liar and use psychodynamic therapy to gain insight into the past of the patient and the reason for lying. It has been found that patients tend to react in a better way to eclectic therapy than other treatment options.

GROUP THERAPY

Group therapy comes along with various advantages. One of the benefits is being a cheaper treatment option as multiple people get treated simultaneously. Also, experts believe that it is much easier to treat a patient group with the same problem as they get a community feeling. People might also opt for treatments that include families, people, and couples. It can work great if the concerned person feels comfortable enough to open up regarding their issues with lying in front of others and looking for connection and accountability. It allows compulsive liars to know how people with the same kind of problem can cope with behavioral issues. It can help in strengthening the system of support for individual patients. In group therapy, situational events might also be practiced where compulsive liars are provided with the needed encouragement for changing their ways.

FAMILY THERAPY

Unfortunately, compulsive lying can result in emotional distress for the family of the liar. Family therapy concentrates on helping the family members to resolve all their conflicts. It can provide them with the needed help to communicate with one another without any need for lies. It might be unavoidable for the family members to blame the compulsive liar for all the family problems. Such families often believe that their family can start functioning normally again by altering the compulsive liar's behaviors. But family therapists encourage every member of the family to collaborate with each other to resolve all sorts of conflicts and not make a compulsive liar feel guilty, as long as they are making progress.

COUPLE THERAPY

It is used for couples who tend to deal with at least one of the members who is a compulsive liar. Couple therapy concentrates on the enhancement of truthful communication between the partners. It can be specifically helpful if one of the partners or both realize that compulsive lying is trying to take a toll on their relationship but still have the faith that their relationship can be saved.

BEFORE THE TREATMENT STARTS

Before opting for the treatment, the concerned person needs to understand and accept that they do have some problem and need treatment. In case they are not cooperative or need to be forced into the treatment, it would be of no help. If that is the case, they are most likely to keep going with their compulsive behaviors and keep lying during the entire course of the treatment.

PROCESS OF TREATMENT

When someone gets treated for excessive lying, the individual is also assessed for some other symptoms or even life situations that might result in their habit of compulsive lying, like neglect or abuse. It helps therapists to treat their dishonesty in the context of their life experiences. As lying itself might turn out to be a symptom for many other disorders, the process of treatment starts with a thorough and careful assessment before moving ahead with any form of treatment. Therapists put into use several observational and interviewing techniques to understand the concerned person as a whole. They are most likely to ask various questions about your present problem, childhood, life experiences, and several other questions. It will help him/her learn about you in detail and start treating your lying problem.

5

SETTING POSITIVE GOALS

The importance of proper goal setting can never be overstated on our journeys in the direction of success. That is why there are so many online articles available today regarding setting positive goals and why it is so important. In the context of compulsive lying, setting positive goals is regarded as a recovery option. Yes, you heard it right. Therapists believe that setting life-enhancing and positive goals will provide you with something you can be genuinely proud of. In this way, deceptive lies and pretentious ego boosts will no longer be needed in the course of life. Learning the necessity of goal setting and the benefits of sticking to the same can act as the defining factor for determining whether we can genuinely embrace the need of setting positive goals. The more you will be willing to embrace this method, the more likely you will reach your definition of personal success, besides dealing with compulsive lying.

WHY IS GOAL SETTING SO IMPORTANT?

Some aspects make goal-setting an essential area of life.

It guides us and aligns our focus

It is pretty hard to reach where you want to in life if you are not sure what exactly you are aiming for. Some people believe that avoiding goals will allow them to live a care-free life. However, is that all that your life has come to? Living a life without plans for avoiding disappointments? When there is no form of a goal in your life, you are most likely to lack a degree of focus and direction. Indeed, you will be able to avoid all kinds of disappointment, but simply by avoiding disappointments, you cannot be happy. In such a case, you are most likely to take the support of lies as you have nothing of yourself. You will try to use the successes of others as yours so that people attend to you. But that won't work.

Without the presence of goals, you will be wasting your energy, efforts, and time. Indeed, talent is necessary; however, all your success will often depend on what you want to do with your talent. What you will be doing with all your talent depends largely on focus. Goals can provide you with direction. You will have something to shoot for. The target and guidance that you develop in your mind will give you the needed help to move toward all your life goals instead of just wandering around aimlessly, telling lies. Plans will help you to align all your behaviors and actions as you keep moving ahead.

It will help you stay away from 'shiny object syndrome'

Shiny object syndrome is always being in pursuit of the

upcoming big thing, continuously switching between goals depending on what makes you feel interesting and the most fun at the moment; however, never providing yourself with time to achieve any of the goals. You won't be able to reach anywhere as you keep changing directions. It is one of the consequences when you decide to live your life without any goal. All your goals, at times, will help in the creation of blinders or mental barriers that will provide you with the needed help to stay focused on all those things that, according to you,are essential and avoid all those things that are of not much priority. As you outline goals, you will be capable of avoiding all those things that tend to distract you from accomplishing all your goals. Setting up goals will help you stay away from the shiny object syndrome as you have developed mental notes that will remind you what you want from life.

Goals will tell you what you want from life and help you realize those things that you need to avoid and give up for achieving the same.

It encourages taking action

Practical goal setting can help in encouraging you to start taking action of all your goals. After all, all your plans will be worthless if you are not willing to give in some effort necessary for executing the same. Setting goals and putting all your plans in place helps bring motivation to start taking action to achieve them. You can write down all your goals and set them somewhere where you can see them all the time. It will provide you with a reminder of all your top priorities. It will also prevent you from getting indulged into lying again.

You can continually improve

It is something that most of the self-improvement and personal development writers talk about – continual improvement. For all those people who are not much aware of the term, continual improvement is about taking small steps in the direction of progress so that you can turn into the person you want to be gradually. The goals you set for yourself will help shape you into the kind of person you want to become. It helps in the shaping of character. All your goals will help in measuring all the progress as you opt for development of this type. Having reasonable goals will help determine the point you started from, your current position, and how further you are required to go. In this way, your goal setting system will act as milestones or benchmarks that will help determine how great you are progressing in the direction of your essential goals.

It helps in keeping you accountable

Goal setting is an excellent way of keeping yourself accountable. Most people fail to reach their goals as they lack the critical aspect of outlining their accountability. For instance, if you set up a plan of doing 100 push-ups, that is a great thing. The majority of people would also support the goal. But the goal lacks accountability. When do you want to opt for the plan, and what steps will you take for the same? These are some of the essential questions that the actual goal leaves unanswered. A much more specific goal would be to opt for 100 push-ups within a timeframe of next four months by starting with ten push-ups and then trying to add five every week. A goal of this nature will help keep you accountable as in case you cannot retain your schedule of progress; you will know that you will not be able to achieve your goal on time.

It will also tell you to reevaluate all those things you are doing and determine the adjustments you will need to succeed.

It can make you feel good

The progress that you can feel and also achieve your goals might turn out to be super addictive and motivating in a good way. The release of dopamine that you get after reaching your goals actsasa small reward for the brain that will inspire you to achieve the next destination. Having some clear and defined plans in possession will provide you with the needed help to feel better regarding yourself and your life in general.

It can help you live the best life

Setting all your goals and defining them clearly will help give you a life that is tailored to your values and beliefs. Your life will get directed in the direction of all those things that you want to achieve. Keep in mind that life is quite a tricky game, and only on rare occasions you will be provided with things on a golden platter. It often needs a great degree of work, proper planning, and effortful execution of both. In simple terms, setting up goals will help you in living a life that will allow you to pursue all your challenges along with rewards that you genuinely want to achieve.

REQUIRED SKILLS FOR GOAL SETTING

Specific skills are necessary for proper goal setting and also achievements. Well, the good news is that they can be developed and learned with practice. In case you fail to achieve the goals that you have set, the main problem may lie in any of these areas:

- **Planning:** Planning of low quality affects the performance negatively in regards to all your goals. Skills of planning and organization can be regarded as integral for the process of goal achievement. With the help of proper planning, you can easily maintain and prioritize concentration on the tasks that you have got in hand while staying away from all sorts of distractions that might draw you away from the final goal.
- **Self-motivation:** Without any desire to achieve, all your attempts at setting goals will be doomed to fail. Having the motivation to attain a goal will allow you to develop new skills and techniques for succeeding. In certain challenging circumstances, the reason to get going is a superb contributor to goal attainment.
- **Management of time:** Time management acts as a great skill across various life sectors and goal setting. Management of time is necessary for the successful accomplishment of goals. In case you fail to consider the timescale needed for achieving a goal, you will inevitably fail. The time that you try to allocate for planning all your goals impacts task performance directly.

- **Self-regulation:** You will need to manage and regulate your own emotions to promote your own social and personal goals.

HELPFUL CATEGORIES TO SET HEALTHY GOALS

When it comes to the context of setting new goals, you can quickly identify the goal type as falling into any of these categories. As you do so, you will get the chance to set new goals in every category or just set more than one goal within each category, permitting your attention to be specific on single or several areas that need attention in particular.

- **Time goals:** You can categorize your goals as long-term or short-term. As the name goes by, short-term goals tend to take lesser time for being achieved rather than long-term goals. Although there is no fixed definition to mark a transition between short-term and long-term goals, you can think of all those goals that will take about one day to a few weeks for achieving as short-term goals and goals to need a minimum of a month as the long-term goals.
- **Focus goals:** They are all about the significant objectives, all those life-changing achievements you are aiming at. All such purposes tend to fall into the category of long-term goals and include steps that need adaptations across several contexts. For instance, if your goal is to write

and publish your first novel within one year, you will need to entail undertaking training about creative writing and also research for self-publishing, a requirement to adjust your current situation of employment for allowing enough time to attain your goal about the dedicated deadline.

- **Topic-based goals:** All such goals tend to fit neatly into a particular life area. Such goals can relate to any aspect of personal life, finances, or your career. For instance, a financial goal might be to save $2,000 within one year, while your personal goal might be to reduce your weight within four months.

The categories of focus, time, and topic are not that exclusive. Instead, all your goals are most likely to come under at least two of the types. Goal setting can act as a great way of having some direction in life to shift all your focus from compulsive lying to achievement of goals. As you get indulged in setting up goals and attaining the same, you won't find any time to get back to your world of lies. So, if you want to deal with your compulsive lying disorder, follow the tips and suggestions from this section and change your life for the good.

❧ 6 ❧

CONSIDERING THE
CONSEQUENCES

Most of us are well adept at lying. All of us lie at times, with ease, small or big, to friends, family members, colleagues, and our loved ones. We tend to lie at times, but they keep lying as a habit when it comes to compulsive liars, as we have already discussed before. Being a compulsive liar is not at all a great thing and also comes with inevitable dangerous consequences that might destroy your life and relationships as well. Sooner or later, a compulsive liar will get exposed, risking people's friendship and trust. However, by admitting all your lies and making sure of a positive change, you can get a second chance of repairing all the broken beliefs. Trust is a fragile thing. Lies and secrets can easily jeopardize trust and might also destroy us along with our relationships. All of us tell 'white lies.' We tend to say, "I am completely fine," when we are not. However, to maintain relationships, you will have to let others know the true you.

Honesty is much more than simply not trying to lie.

Deception involves making vague or ambiguous statements, manipulating information using emphasis, opting for half-truths, minimizing or exaggerating, and withholding information or feelings essential for someone who comes with the right to know. Lies can effectively affect relationships and friendships and also deprives others of informed action and freedom of choice. Let us have a look at some of the consequences of compulsive lying so that you can start treating the same as soon as possible for your betterment.

THE REAL COST OF LYING

The majority of people who opt for lies tend to worry about the risk of being honest; however, they give little or no thought to the linked risks of dishonesty. Some of the definite ways in which lying can result in harm are:

- They tend to block true intimacy among partners. Intimacy is wholly based on authenticity and trust. When someone comes to find out that their partner or friend is lying to them without any reason, it can affect the relationship significantly.
- They can result in omissions and cover-up lies that might be tough to remember. All of these tend to mount up, and in case the truth somehow comes out, it might hurt more even than the actual lie. The longer someone lies, the harder will be the hurdle of revelation. It would bring up the question of every instance

of covering up and all the times that the innocent other person trusted and relied upon the liar.

- Honesty gets valued as a moral norm, though the specifics and context might differ among cultures. As someone tries to violate cultural or religious standards by lying, they tend to experience anxiety generated by guilt. Despite the best efforts of dishonesty, the physiological reactions are the basis for electronic lie detectors.

- The violation of values not only results in guilt but also affects our self-concept. Over a long time, deception can slowly eat away our self-esteem. The ordinary nature of the responsibility that could have been reversed with honesty now turns into shame. Also, it undermines the fundamental sense of worthiness and dignity as an individual. The prevalent gap between the way we feel inside and show others tends to widen.

- The ways of managing shame and guilt result in more problems. Compulsive liars not only hide the secret but more of who they are. Liars might opt for resentments to justify their actions, become critical, aggressive, or irritable. They tend to rationalize all their lies or secrets to avoid any form of inner conflict. Some people tend to get so obsessed with their lies that they face difficulties concentrating on other things.

- Lying results in mental distress, along with various health complaints.
- The victim might start reacting to avoidance behaviors from others by feeling anxious, angry, confused, needy, suspicious, or abandoned. They might begin to doubting themselves, while their level of self-esteem might also suffer.

WHEN YOU LIE, YOUR BRAIN GETS OVERWHELMED

The very second a lie comes out of your mouth, your body starts releasing cortisol in your brain. After a few moments, your mind goes into overdrive while trying to remember the truth and the lie. At such a point, decision-making might turn out to be a challenging task, and you might also opt for projecting all your discomfort in the form of anger. All of this happens within the first ten minutes of lying.

YOUR LEVEL OF STRESS INCREASES

After the initial reactions, you might start feeling worried about the lie or about getting caught. To deal with such a feeling, you might opt to treat the other person in a kinder way than you usually do. After lying, one of these might happen if you are a compulsive liar, you might start believing the lie. In case you are not a compulsive liar, you might still have bad feelings and try to stay away from the person you lied to. All of these sums up to extra stress that comes with various other negative consequences on your overall health. It might enhance your level of blood pressure, lower back pain, cause headaches, and reduce the count of your white blood cells. Remember that a significant amount of energy goes into developing a lie and telling the same. It might slowly result in depression and anxiety. It does not even stop there as all such feelings might also affect your digestion process, resulting in cramps and nausea.

IT CAN WEAR YOU OUT EMOTIONALLY

While all of it might not feel like anything significant at the moment, the problem with lies is that they need continuous maintenance. In case you even tell a tiny lie once, you will have to remember the same for a long time for maintaining the story. All of it might seem like a very exhausting charade, specifically when you tell one lie to every person in your life and all of them come together for a party at your place. In case the lie is not that significant, it might not have this kind of effect; however, when you know that the information might come up again, it will be best for you to stick to the truth.

LIES MIGHT KEEP YOU AWAY FROM ADDRESSING THE ACTUAL ISSUE

When telling lies, it is an essential thing to ask yourself why exactly you are doing it. No matter if you can admit the same to yourself or not, lies always act as a way of putting covers on a more profound truth. In place of paying attention to the actual issue, being fully honest with your close ones, or uncovering some of the facts in therapy, lies come with the capability of piling up more problems on the plate. Well, all of that can easily make the overall situation worse for you.

THEY TEND TO TAKE A TOLL ON YOUR RELATIONSHIPS

It is an essential thing to keep in mind is that lies might feel as if they are preserving all your relationships. However, in actuality, they will be doing the exact opposite. Each lie keeps separating the understanding of compulsive liars of who they are from who they think they are. In case you are not comfortable with discussing something, you can keep it as it is. But if you keep hiding things and telling lies to your loved ones, it might readily affect all your relationships, and thus making you feel alienated at a later time.

LIES ARE EQUAL TO ANXIETY

With all kinds of covering-ups and maintenance going on, there is nothing to wonder that lies can easily result in the sense of anxiety. When you keep worrying about getting caught, you might develop feelings of panic. Well, the funny thing is that most of us tend to lie to prevent our anxious feelings. So, correctly understanding that they might enhance your feelings of anxiety is a great thing to remember.

LIES CAN MAKE YOU FEEL ISOLATED

In place of just relaxing and enjoying the course of life, lies demand you all the time to keep a continuous list of all those people who knows what, and also what you said to each one of those people. Well, all of this might turn out to be excessively isolating. When you face challenging times remembering all your false stories and maintaining things straight, you might feel the urge to stay away from engaging with other people. After all, it will be a lot easier for you to just chill with yourself, rather than going out, telling a lie, and risk getting caught up. In case you find yourself in a similar situation, setting up records might work the best for you.

LYING AFFECTS SLEEPING PATTERN

Because of all kinds of anxieties involved, lies can easily keep you awake the whole night. As you keep lying or suffer from compulsive lying disorder, you might face problems with your sleep patterns because of excessive worrying regarding maintaining your stories straight. Besides making you feel dizzy and tired, lack of sleep can easily make way to some other chronic mental health issues, like depression, anxiety, and many others. In such a case, opening your heart out to a therapist or a mental health expert might work as the safest bet for you. It will also help you uncover the root of all your lies and the reason behind it.

THEY MIGHT RESULT IN TRUST ISSUES

Keeping aside the point of whether others come to find out that you are lying or not, by opting for simple lies, you will be developing issues of trust with yourself and with other people as well. As you lie, no matter whether you are conscious of the same or not, you send a message to others and yourself that neither can handle the feelings that come along with the truth. The ultimate result of this is that you will start trusting yourself less, besides trusting others less.

LYING MIGHT RESULT IN A SENSE OF INSECURITY

Telling only a small number of lies can quickly develop feelings of insecurity. There is a definite reason why this happens. As safety and trust tend to go hand-in-hand, the overall effect of telling lies, with time, is a deep-seated fear of insecurity that can easily affect all your relationships – romantic, platonic, and professional. To put it in simple terms, you are most likely to start feeling insecure every time you lie.

LYING LOWERS SELF-ESTEEM

Telling a small lie for keeping someone happy, like telling your wife that you loved the food she cooked for you, is okay. However, when you opt for lies for covering up something important to yourself or opt for lying as you cannot address the truth, it might negatively impact. Lying habitually can easily hamper personality traits, and as you know that you cannot be honest, you might start thinking less of yourself. The guilt you feel for misleading other people might cause you to start second-guessing the type of person you are.

LYING MIGHT MAKE YOU FEEL MISUNDERSTOOD

For getting people to treat you the way you want to be treated, and for people to understand you, you are required to be honest. So, there is nothing to feel surprised that you start feeling misunderstood right after telling a lie. As you opt for lies, you deliver other people around you with a false impression of yourself and what you are going through. If you tend to lie to your boss, friends, and others about the extent to which you can deal with emotional health, they might falsely assume that stacking up more on you or having greater expectations from you is entirely acceptable. When you fail to deliver or just fall short, they might take your failures personally or have no form of empathy for you. It might slowly take the form of a vicious cycle.

Compulsive lying is a disorder that needs to be taken proper care of, especially after analyzing all the consequences that it might lead to. Try to determine all your lies and start working on them right now for a better life ahead.

᪥ 7 ᪥
HOW TO STOP LYING IN A
RELATIONSHIP?

One single lie comes with the power of shattering years of hard-earned trust. Consistently lying to your romantic partner will result in the downfall of your relationship. If you truly value your partner and still keep up your dishonesty regarding all your deeds and feelings, you are left with two options – either stop the cycle of lies or just end the relationship itself. Can you face a situation where your romantic partner stops trusting you? Can you stand the risk of losing your partner completely? What's worse, if you tend to be a compulsive liar, you might not even get any kind of respect from your partner. Even when you get separated, your future will be doomed because you were obsessed with lying one after the other. In case you think that you are not able to stop lying, and if you feel your life is heading towards a miserable state, you must opt for professional help.

It will always be better for you to start working on dealing with your lies before you lose your partner completely.

BELIEVING AND TRUSTING YOUR PARTNER

Well, this suggestion might sound weird as you are the one who is lying. However, people tend to lie when they cannot trust the person they are lying to. For example, you might opt for lying about your real feelings regarding your partner's family as you are afraid that your partner might dismiss what you say immediately and just side with their family. You might opt to lie about yourself as you cannot trust your romantic partner enough to share the truth of your troubled past. No matter what is the reaction of your partner, you should believe and trust him/her. Without trust, you won't be able to be honest, and it can be said that your relationship will never have a stable footing.

BEING TRUSTWORTHY

Indeed, you can never start trusting your partner when you are not that trustworthy. It is not a far cry to state that the only reason people tend to lie is that they are trying to hide something indecent or immoral. If you are not willing to lie to your partner about cheating, it will be better to not get engaged in any affair. If you are not willing to lie regarding spending all the joint account savings on gambling, then stop wasting both of your money. It is as simple as that. As you start being trustworthy, you can quickly eliminate the problem from even existing.

COUNTING TO FIVE AND TELLING THE TRUTH

Now, in case you have done something terrible already, such as cheating on your romantic partner, you will need to count till five and just confront the truth. The countdown of five seconds is long enough for getting yourself prepared for that moment; however, it is short enough to prevent yourself from overthinking or just moving back. You have opted for something wrong, and the least that can be done on your part is to admit the same to your partner. The longer you try to hide the truth, and the longer you deny, the problem will last longer, and the overall consequences will be much more complex. So, right before it gets too late, go for the countdown and just tell the truth. It will just cut off the necessity to lie any further, and it might also bring back trust in the relationship.

PRACTICING OPEN COMMUNICATION

For being truly honest with one another, both your partner and you need to opt for open communication consistently. When you tell your partner what you feel and think and do the same in return, you will understand and be comfortable with each other. It will help in discarding the compulsion to lie and hide things. It is only when you start communicating with each other the relationship becomes genuine. It will be free from the shackles of apprehension and deceit.

EMPATHIZING WITH YOUR PARTNER

In case you constantly find yourself lying to your romantic partner, try to imagine the opposite as well. What would you feel when you determine the truth? You might feel disrespected, betrayed, and in some cases of extreme nature, defiled. Right? Surely no one wants to be lied to and just make a fool of themselves. Try to use empathy as the shield to stop you from attaching the blades of lies against your romantic partner.

LOOKING FOR A PARTNER WHOM YOU TRULY LOVE AND VALUE

It can be regarded as more of a dramatic measure. In case you constantly find yourself lying to your romantic partner, without thinking of the pain that it might cause to him/her for the long-term, then you might just not love or value him/her as much you think. At such a point, it would be a responsibility of yours to end the relationship. It is the only way in which you can stop lying indeed. You will have to spare both of you the trouble of being in a relationship with constant lies. Try to look for someone who you genuinely care for and value enough not to lie to. But right before you opt for a new partner, try to take note of all those items included here to stop yourself from repeating the same mistake.

REMOVING LYING FROM LIFESTYLE

Even when you consider the items of the previous suggestion and try to opt for a person you love and value truly, if
lying tends to be a regular part of your lifestyle, then the
chances are high that you might end up lying over again.
When you keep lying to everyone every day, lying will
automatically turn out to be a habit. It takes the shape of a
natural impulse where you are most likely to be desensi-
tized to the detrimental effects. So, you will have to
provide some sincere effort to remove continuous lying
from your daily life first. As you do so, you will not only be
able to be more honest with your partner, but it will also
turn you into a better person altogether.

KNOWING THE GAP BETWEEN BAD LIES AND GOOD LIES

Not all lies can be regarded to be wrong. There are all
those that are acceptable, depending on the situation and
the frequency of use. But you need to tell the difference to
avoid any kind of confusion regarding a terrible lie as the
good one. A great example of a good lie is when you try to
say that you enjoyed your partner's cooking, even though
it was full of salt. You do so to show appreciation to your
partner and not make them feel wrong about the dish they
made for you for hours. In a situation of this nature, of
course, context is essential. If your partner cooked for you
as she wanted to give a surprise to you, then it is all okay
to say that you very much loved the dish. But if your
partner wanted you to taste the dish as he/she is going for

a cooking competition or if they expressly tell you to provide honest feedback, then you must inform the truth.

A great example of a bad lie is saying that you will come back late as you have a late-night meeting at the office when in actuality, you had some late-night love affair. No matter the nature of the context, a lie of this nature can never be accepted. But you will have to avoid bad lies and keep practicing with caution while making the good ones. Trust is an essential component needed for a long-lasting relationship. Lies tend to act like the arch enemies of honesty and trust. So, both you and your partner must keep doing all those things that can help avoid lies and prevent lies from corrupting the state of your relationship. Practice good lies, keeping aside the bad ones.

ACCEPTING YOUR FAULT

You will have to stop convincing yourself that your way is the only best way. You might have your set of reasons to lie to your partner whom you love. But it is a common thing to wish to convince yourself that you are never wrong as you lie. Your inner critic is always in the process of justifying all your lies. The only fact that your partner might be disrespecting you, neglecting you, or even takes you for granted is because you keep lying to him/her. But you will have to understand that all such wrongdoings should never justify all your lies which is also wrong. Can you feel better about opting for the wrong path? Indeed, you would not feel better. Try to be honest to yourself first, and you will come to see that your tendency to lie to your partner will also decrease.

RESPECTING YOURSELF

The very moment you start respecting yourself, you will come to understand the value of your own words. You can understand what it means to be in the position that others tend to point their fingers at you. As you start understanding your true worth, you will withhold yourself from some embarrassing situation. So, respect is something that you will have to cultivate with time. Liars are not aware of how their actions tend to affect their image. At times, all they enjoy is manipulating others to get the best out of any situation.

SEEING THINGS FROM THE POINT OF VIEW OF YOUR PARTNER

As you start thinking about the person you are lying to, you can empathize more with the precarious position of that person. Would you ever want to be in a position where you are not even aware of the truth? Would you like to have several things happening behind you, specifically if you are the one who is at the receiving end of all the lies? No one would ever want to be in such a position. As you start lying to your partner, you will slowly lose trust. All of us deserve to be aware of what is happening in various situations that directly affect our lives.

ANALYZING THE ROOT CAUSE

You know it very well. Lying can never be worthy of all the sufferings that you will have to go through. If you are willing to give up lying, you will have to analyze the root cause that you keep lying all the time. Are you having some other kind of issues? Is help required? Has your habit of lying turned out to be a threat to others? These are some of the questions you will have to analyze right before you make up your mind about the root cause.

ROAD TO RECOVERY

Even all those who have learned how to overcome all their negative behaviors might develop sheer feelings of guilt right after analyzing the kind of damage they have done to people around them. All of this might position a huge burden on the shoulders of a person. That individual might never recover from the overall effects of compulsive lying fully if they fail to learn how to forgive themselves. There are some important concepts that are essential for recovery. Let's have a look at them.

BEING ACCOUNTABLE FOR ALL THE ACTIONS

Accountability is one thing that most people expect from others who do not always tell the truth. After you recognize that compulsive lying might result in hurting others or even yourself, you will have to remember that you have got full control over all your choices. It indicates that when you decide to opt for a lie, you will also have to make yourself ready for the consequences of the actions.

PRACTICE APOLOGIZING

The moment you find yourself telling a lie, try to correct your statement as fast as possible, even if it needs changing the entire story. It will help you in being more apologetic and also truthful. There is nothing to worry about what others think of you – your loved ones and your friends can understand you in a better way if you try to tell them that your story is not as great as you thought it should be. Doing so will allow them to be better aware of the situation and accept you for who you are. Keep in mind that you can never predict what is going on inside the mind of another person. While it is normal for some people to voice out their frustration or look surprised as you keep telling the truth, you will have to remember that all these are natural and normal reactions. It is most likely that others will try to brush off any mistake you make or simply laugh it off. You can start feeling better as you find out that nothing bad or terrible will happen as you tell the truth.

LEARNING TO FORGIVE YOURSELF

Forgiving your self is one of the important and the most difficult part of recovery. As you start trusting the truth that you can be the person who you are, and there no exists no form of pressure for you to be the person that others want you to be, you will come to realize that accepting that you can make mistakes will let you improve yourself. There will be times when you might feel that you are not in control. However, that happens to all of us. In case you feel that things should have taken place differently and you might have acted differently as well, just let it go. If you feel that others might not be that kind to you if you start being true to yourself, then try to exert the same kind of kindness to your self instead. Most of the factors involved in you turning into a compulsive liar were not within your control. You will have to keep in mind that you are giving the best now, and that is all that matters in the present day, tomorrow, and for the remaining part of your life.

MEDITATING AND REFLECTING

Meditation can be considered a great tool for the process of personal healing and also for the enhancement of self-awareness. You might not get the chance to alter the past; however, you can certainly do something good for the future. There are several forms of meditation, and all of them involve only one thing – not withholding your feelings. With the help of meditation, you will get the chance to be more in the present, without any kind of anxiety that might arise in your modern life, besides learning how you can channel your focus and energy. Try to set aside a minimum of ten minutes every day for meditation. Start by taking deep breaths and let your guilt feelings and frustration come out. You will aim to properly realize that guilt is a kind of feeling that tends to come along only with compulsive lying. It cannot dictate who you are as a human being. Try to notice the rising feelings; however, try not to get attached to them so that they can get the chance of defining your behavior.

ATONEMENT

The guilt that any compulsive liar feels is their way of atoning to their lies. In place of just feeling miserable, try to channel the same energy and opt for some therapeutic work, like volunteering for charities.

DOING THINGS THAT INSPIRE YOU

Try and make a list of all those things that tend to give you a happy feeling. Do one thing that truly makes you happy as the reward of not lying, whether it is going out for a run, meditation, or as simple as reading a book. As you opt for pleasurable things that do not include lying will help create positive reinforcement for you. It might also turn out to be a great idea if you start doing all those things that you liked originally. For example, if you loved riding bicycles in your past days and now you pretend to like cars, it is your chance of getting back to the old hobby. Simply by acknowledging that you can also like things without any need for other's approval, you can start discovering things that you enjoy about yourself. At the same time, you can start with information and accomplishments in all those fields you are really good in. As you do so, you will get the awareness that you can truly feel happy as you tell your real achievements, in place of the ones that you tend to make up as you keep flowing in the momentum of any conversation.

SUBLIMINAL MESSAGE FOR HONESTY

Watching and listening to subliminal messages that are created for compulsive liars can be very helpful. As you subject yourself to repeated messages, you would not be aware of all the alterations within your subconscious. It can act as a great way for brain rewiring. The best way of doing this is to setthe alarm for every hour or after every few hours, and when the alarm goes off, you will have to read a message to yourself. Your brain will soon start noticing this pattern and will also help in speeding up the entire process. For instance, a message that you can read to yourself is, "Everything that I say has value as it generates from me, and not because I need the approval of others." One more example – "My failures or achievements cannot determine who I am. The way I treat other people and my character define who I am."

In case you are facing issues with feelings of shame or guilt, keep in mind that compulsive lying is more like an addiction and cannot be regarded as a moral issue. As you adopt this mindset, you can prevent yourself from getting too down on yourself. You can never be a bad person only for having some kind of detrimental behavioral flaw. Also, it is quite essential to realize that several other factors are not within your control and caused you to opt for the behavioral trait in the very first place.

THINKING CAREFULLY RIGHT BEFORE YOU SPEAK

Carefully thinking before you speak is an effective and straightforward technique. You will need to ensure that when someone presents you with some question that you are inclined to answer, pause for a moment, and think about that answer you are willing to give. If you do not feel like answering the question with some true statement, you will have to ensure that you are aware of the false statement you want to give. You will have to be sure that you consciously choose what is false and what is true, besides why and why not, you made up your mind to opt for the truth in some situations. Also, you might start feeling self-conscious as you take some time to get into a conversation in the first place; however, you will have to keep in mind that you are doing this for the long-term effect. You can try to practice consciously thinking about all those things you are about to say right before you speak.

Remind yourself consistently during the day to take deep breaths and give your statements a thought before speaking up. As you start affirming this to yourself, you will be less likely to lie impulsively when presented with a question. Another useful tip that can help you in this new practice is to start thinking that the lungs are lowering down right into the pelvis as you breathe deeply. As you try to incorporate this form of deep breathing into your regular life, you can notice that nervousness and panic will dissipate, thus, permitting you to start communicating without much fear. If you speak, try to talk slower and add more pauses as you talk, specifically when you are talking or speaking about those topics that you are not much comfortable with. It will allow you to be conscious of all your behaviors, and the effect will surely surprise you.

OPT FOR JOURNALING

You will have to record all the lies, along with the hard truths, that you opt for telling every day. Explore the circumstances surrounding all those behaviors, besides the setting, your emotional state, the time, and many other aspects. As you constantly do this, you will begin recognizing the triggers and patterns of all your behaviors. You might realize that you start being dishonest as you get stressed or when someone specific is present around you. Right from there, you can start working on why you tend to act in that way and how you can improve such situations in the future. As you keep journaling, you will need to clarify the aspects of your life that you want to be honest about. Try to set the same in proper order.

You can start by delving deeper into the aspects of your life that you least and most confident about, along with the aspects that you are least and most honest about. You will have to give your best to be as specific as possible. Keep in mind that journaling can be done in plenty of ways, and it all depends on you how little or how much you want to do. However, there are some principles to guide you in the process. Try to see every truth and lie as important. Do not allow small lies to pass by. You can keep a personal standard of being truthful in every aspect of your life. You will have to view all your small lies pass like an avalanche that will slowly compound over time if you fail to notice the same at the right time.

AFTERWORD

Thank you for making it through to the end of the *Compulsive Lying Mastery*; let's hope it was very informative and was able to provide you with all of the necessary tools you need to reach your goals, whatever they may be.

I have given my best to gather all the possible strategies in this guidebook to help a compulsive liar deal with his/her lying problems. One thing that can be guaranteed is that if you try to be consistent, all the strategies you can find in this book will surely work. Try to be a bit optimistic regarding your present situation, and keep making small changes every passing day. Keep in mind that all of us struggle with our issues. Some people come with a gambling addiction, some face difficulties opting for a healthy diet, and others come with physical disabilities. What is essential to note that nobody is better inherently in comparison to others.

There is nothing to feel inferior about suffering from low self-esteem or compulsive lying. Try to have a long-term perspective and just concentrate on the kind of person you can become. You will see that things will start working out as you want them to. So, have faith in yourself and opt for the required change. I wish you good luck on the journey.

www.ingramcontent.com/pod-product-compliance
Lightning Source LLC
Chambersburg PA
CBHW022105020426
42335CB00012B/839